Reinaldo Vázquez Oliva
Rosío De La Caridad Estrada Fonseca
Osvaldo Amador Aguiar

Ischemic heart disease

Reinaldo Vázquez Oliva
Rosío De La Caridad Estrada Fonseca
Osvaldo Amador Aguiar

Ischemic heart disease

Risk factors associated with older adults.

ScienciaScripts

Imprint

Cover image: www.ingimage.com

This book is a translation from the original published under ISBN 978-613-9-40562-6.

Publisher:
Sciencia Scripts
is a trademark of
Dodo Books Indian Ocean Ltd. and OmniScriptum S.R.L publishing group

120 High Road, East Finchley, London, N2 9ED, United Kingdom
Str. Armeneasca 28/1, office 1, Chisinau MD-2012, Republic of Moldova, Europe
Printed at: see last page
ISBN: 978-620-7-74397-1

EXERGO

``…The doctor be something further that someone that attends to one that HE sick and goes to hospital, but that will have a paper special in the medicine preventive, …, in end, be a << Guardian of the Health >>´´. (1983)

Fidel Castro Ruz

DEDICATION

I dedicate this job:

- *TO my children,Alexandra,Alessandra,Danny my elderly treasure, by be my inspiration and the force that drives my days.*
- *TO my wife Gleibis by his love and by be my unconditional support .*
- *TO my parents Gisela and Raphael by always help me .*
- *TO all the that they trusted in that could arrive to the final.*

ACKNOWLEDGEMENT

I appreciate:

- *Me family in special to my parents because fill my life of reasons to continue fighting.*
- *To the Revolution that gave me the opportunity for my professional improvement and make my dreams come true.*
- *TO my Tutor by his aid in this stage so important of my life.*
- *TO the friendships that I they helped and that always they trusted in my.*

SUMMARY

Cardiovascular diseases are among the main causes of death in the world. Ischemic heart disease is one of the main health problems in the elderly, its incidence follows an ascending curve and presents a high mortality, with the objective of determining the risk factors associated with ischemic heart disease in older adults, from office 8 of the Manacas health area During 2019, a case AND control study was carried out. The case group was made up of 34 older adults with a diagnosis of ischemic heart disease and was matched 1:1 according to sex to the controls. Statistical analysis was performed by percentage method and odds ratio. It turned out that 61.7% of the cases belonged to the male sex and 79.5% were over 70 years old, angina was found in 47%; A 5-fold higher probability of developing heart disease was identified in patients with a history of ischemic heart disease in first-degree relatives, 2 times more in smokers, 12 times more in diabetics, 23 times more in hypertensive patients, 15 times more in patients with dyslipidemia and approximately 6 times more in obese people. Ischemic heart disease in Adults office seniors 8 of the Manacas area predominate in male patients and increases directly proportional to age. Angina is the most common. All the factors studied behaved as predisposing factors for the development of heart disease, high blood pressure, dyslipidemia and diabetes mellitus stand out in that order.

.

INDEX

INTRODUCTION

Background from the description of Coronary heart disease dates back to The people who occupied Mesopotamia where the heart was considered the center of the movements of the soul, within a theocratic medicine, deeply religious and practiced by priests, during the splendor of the Egyptian civilization is described in the Ebers papyrus, which was Myocardial infarction found in the tomb of THEBES

``... Yeah examine still man because this sick of the heart and has pains in the arms, in he chest and in a side stand of his heart... death threatens him ...´´
In Greece, the works attributed to Hippocrates contain many clinical descriptions on the subject where he describes the characteristics and irradiation of cardiac pain. (1)

When we say myocardial infarction, it currently refers to cardiac cell death due to ischemia due to an imbalance in perfusion demand. (2)

Ischemic heart disease in older adults is more likely than in younger people. Aging can cause changes in the heart and blood vessels that can increase a person's risk of developing cardiovascular disease. Its most common change is increased stiffness of the major arteries, called arteriosclerosis (3) . Cardiovascular diseases are the leading cause of death in this sector; in the elderly, the clinical presentation is usually atypical, with acute non-ST elevation myocardial infarction being more common. (4)

Myocardial infarction, for its part, is the most frequent presentation of ischemic heart disease. The World Health Organization estimated that in 2012, 12.6% of deaths worldwide were due to ischemic heart disease that is the main cause of death in developed countries and the third cause of death in developing countries, after AIDS and lower respiratory infections. (5)

In developed countries like the UNITED STATES, deaths from heart disease outnumber deaths from cancer. The Coronary artery disease causes one in 5 deaths in the United States and where more than one million people suffer a coronary attack each year, of which 40% will die as a result of the heart attack. So one American will die every minute from a pathological coronary event. (6

In India, cardiovascular disease is the leading cause of death. In this country, a third of deaths during 2007 were due to cardiovascular disease, a figure that is expected to increase from one million in 2020 and 1.6 million in 2025, to two million by 2030 (7)

In Europe, cardiovascular diseases are the leading cause of death between men and women, being responsible almost the half of deaths (42%). They are also the main cause of disability and decrease in quality of life. Although there are important divergences between European countries in the prevalence figures of cardiovascular diseases and the impact and evolution of the different risk factors, the problem is common in all the countries. (8) In Spain, as in he rest of the In countries of the

Mediterranean area, mortality from cardiovascular disease is half of that observed in the countries of northern Europe and USA and a third of that observed in Eastern European countries, even so, cardiovascular diseases being the main cause of death and illness (9)

In 2002, they caused 125,797 deaths, which represents 34% of all deaths (30% in men and 39% in women). However, by sex, only in women is cardiovascular disease the first cause of death (in men it is the second, after tumors), and by specific groups of age, cardiovascular diseases are the first cause of death only after 70 years of age, ranking in second position, behind tumors, in middle-aged people. (10)

In Mexico, heart diseases have been the leading cause of death for 20 years and among them, ischemic heart disease accounts for 41.9 percent of the total annual deaths due to heart diseases. heart. (eleven)

In Chile it is the main cause of death and age is one of the main factors associated with mortality, which leads to mortality in older adult patients being even higher. (12)

It is estimated that in 2017, 18.1 million people died from this cause, of which 80% lived in low- and middle-income countries. (13)

In 2017, 1.5 million deaths from cardiovascular disease occurred in the Americas, in America Latin and He Caribbean the disease of the heart t represents 31% of the total deaths, predominating the age group of 65 years and over. (14)

In Ecuador, cardiovascular diseases occupy first place among the causes of mortality and among them myocardial infarction. Its incidence is close to 40,000 people a year, which means that every 12 minutes an Ecuadorian suffers a heart attack (15).

Ischemic heart disease and particularly myocardial infarction is the number one cause of cardiovascular mortality in the adult population of Venezuela. In Venezuela, ischemic heart disease is responsible for 31,338 deaths annually, that is, 18% of all mortality and 58% of mortality due to cardiovascular disease (16).

In Cuba, despite the introduction of streptokinase and the integrated medical emergency system, in the 1990s myocardial infarction continues to have a notable impact on the health of the population; since 1940, cardiovascular diseases have topped the death statistics., represents the first cause of death in both sexes, with an average of 11.5 years of life potentially lost as consequence of the disease (17). In Cuba in 2016, heart diseases occupied the first cause of death With a total Of 24,462 deaths, 66.05% were due to ischemic diseases and of these 44.42 were due to myocardial infarction. The provinces with the highest incidence were Havana, Santiago de Cuba Matanzas, Holguín and Villa Clara, occupying in 2016 the mortality by diseases of the heart he second place in the groups of fifteen- 49 years and 50-64 years, as well as the first place after 65 years (18). Ischemic heart diseases caused a total of 16,435 deaths during that period, for a rate of 146.43 per 100,000 inhabitants, and of these, 7,022 were caused by myocardial infarction (19). The mortality rate from cardiovascular diseases has increased from 148.2 per 100,000 inhabitants in 1970 to 241.6 in 2017 (20) .

According to data published in the 2020 Health Yearbook in Cuba, in 2018 there were 25 766 deaths by disease cardiovascular while that in 2019 the number rose to 26,736 (21)

In Villa Clara in 2016 the crude death rate from ischemic heart disease exceeded the national rate. In the same period of time in Villa Clara, 2,716 people died from cardiovascular diseases. The municipality of Santa Clara occupies one of the first places in deaths from ischemic heart disease, related to multiple risk factors and age, which It serves as one of the most important, because it is the province with the greatest aging population in the country (22). In Santo Domingo in 2019 the The second cause of death was heart disease with a rate of 218.4% per 10,000 inhabitants, predominating the age group 75 years and older, acting as one of the main causes of death in the town of Manaca (23).

Despite advances in the treatment of acute myocardial infarction, impact of preventive measures is offset by the alarming increase of the obesity, the hypertension arterial, the diabetes mellitus he aging of the population and the appearance of other comorbidities, such as kidney failure. (24)

Control of risk factors is an essential element for the primary and secondary prevention of cardiovascular diseases. These interact with each other, in such a way that the sum of several of them has a multiplicative effect on the overall risk. The best tool to establish Priority in primary cardiovascular prevention is the accurate estimation of cardiovascular risk. (25)

Knowledge of the risk factors, as well as their magnitude, represents a great advance for a better understanding of this cardiac pathology and in this way propose impact strategies to reduce its incidence and its consequences, and irreversible such as mortality. (26)

Scientific problem :

For all of the above, we are motivated to carry out this research to answer the question: What are the risk factors associated with ischemic heart disease in older adults in CMF No. 8 of the Manacas polyclinic, in the period 2019-2020 ?

GOALS

GENERAL:

Determine the factors of risk associated to the heart disease ischemic in the older adult in the period 2019-2020 in CMF No 8 of the Manacas polyclinic

SPECIFICS:

1. Describe he cluster of cases according to variables clinical epidemiological of interest
2. Compare both groups according to factors of risk of ischemic heart disease

THEORETICAL FRAMEWORK

The increase in prevalence and hospitalizations for heart failure in developed countries in recent decades makes ischemic heart disease one of the cardiovascular epidemics of the 21st century. Cuba is a developing country, however, many of its health indicators are close to developed ones. Its population is very aged, in 1999 22.8% of the total were 50 and over and 13% were 60 and over, which increases the occurrence of cardiovascular diseases. The Cuban health profile is characterized by the predominance of chronic non-communicable diseases among the leading causes of mortality. For more than 40 years, heart diseases have topped health statistics as the main cause of death, including heart disease. ischemic that is a of the first Causes of death in Cuba 'responsible for one in four deaths in the country and represents almost 80% of all deaths from heart disease in both sexes. (27)

Historically, ischemia has been defined as tissue anemia (absence of red blood cells) due to obstruction of arterial flow. Myocardial ischemia is characterized by an imbalance between the demand and supply of oxygen to the myocardium (28)

When the mechanism of ischemia is a deficit in the supply of oxygen, it is called supply ischemia. It occurs when there is a reduction in arterial blood flow due to obstruction of a coronary artery (formation of a thrombus, stenosis) or due to increased coronary vascular tone (vasospasm). This situation HE associate with frequency to syndromes coronary sharp. The Myocardial ischemia may also be caused by hypoxia, when oxygen delivery is reduced despite adequate blood flow and tissue perfusion. This occurs in cases of asphyxiation, carbon monoxide poisoning, congenital heart disease cyanotic either anemia serious, among others. (29)

On the other hand, in the presence of severe chronic coronary obstruction with relatively fixed coronary blood flow, an increase in oxygen demand, usually due to exercise or emotion, may produce an insufficient increase in coronary blood flow and produce demand ischemia. (29)

Causes of the myocardial ischemia
Coronary artery disease is due in the vast majority of cases to an obstruction of the coronary arteries by atheromatous plaques. (30)

Disease coronary different of atherosclerosis
Arteritis - Luetics - Granulomatous - Polyarteritis nodes - Kawasaki - Lupus erythematosus - Rheumatoid arthritis Coronary trauma, radiotherapy

Disease metabolic with slimming coronary - Mucopolysaccharidosis - Homocysteinuria - Fabry disease - Amyloidosis - Juvenile intimal sclerosis

Narrowing luminal by others mechanisms - Dissection coronary - Dissection of aorta - Coronary spasm

Coronary embolism - Infective endocarditis - Mitral prolapse - Prosthetic valve embolism - Mixona - Embolism paradoxical - Associate to surgery coronary Anomaly congenital coronary Imbalance between oxygen supply and demand - Aortic stenosis - Aortic insufficiency - Carbon monoxide poisoning - Takotsubo - Thyrotoxicosis - Prolonged hypotension

Hematological disease - Polycythemia Vera - Thrombocytosis - Dismeminated intravascular coagulation Miscellany - Abuse of cocaine - Contusion myocardial - Iatrogenic (32)

An episode of severe ischemia can produce prolonged myocardial dysfunction with a gradual return of contractile activity, a condition called stunned myocardium. Stunned myocardium is represented by persistent regional dysfunction when chest pain, ST segment shift, and regional perfusion have recovered. In patients with myocardial infarction, the stunned myocardium is adjacent to the infarcted one. Improvement in ventricular dysfunction occurs gradually over days to weeks. Stunned myocardium is also characteristic of unstable angina (33)

Impaired left ventricular function at rest due to a chronic reduction in blood flow that can be restored by revascularization is attributed to a hibernating myocardium. Even some akinetic segments can sometimes recover systolic contraction after revascularization. Is It is possible to identify dysfunctional hibernated myocardium with non-invasive methods such as echocardiography, perfusion scintigraphy and magnetic resonance imaging.

This has relevant practical importance because revascularization can improve the function ventricular left, relieve the symptoms of insufficiency cardiac, in the long term, avoid myocardial necrosis. Myocardial necrosis is defined as myocardial cell death secondary to sustained ischemia. The subendocardium is the most sensitive region because its energy needs, metabolism, and oxygen extraction rate are higher. Severely ischemic myocardium undergoes necrosis that begins in the subendocardium 15 to 20 minutes after coronary artery occlusion. Necrosis advances towards the epicardium like a wave, gradually affecting the outer epicardial layers with a lower degree of ischemia. Wave progression is slowed by the presence of residual blood flow when coronary obstruction is incomplete or when mature collaterals exist at the time of obstruction. In acute coronary obstruction, the subendocardial lateral limits of the subendocardial infarction are established in the first hour, while the myocardial infarction increases in a transmural direction for 4 to 6 hours. This observation of time-dependent progression of necrosis is the rationale for timely interventions to salvage the myocardium. (3. 4)

The Spanish Association of Cardiology proposes that ischemic heart disease, according to the forms of presentation, can be classified into

Syndrome chronic coronary
•Agina stable chronic
• Microvascular agina

•Ischemia silent

Syndrome coronary sharp
•With ascent persistent of the S.T. heart attack sharp of myocardium transmural
• Without ascent persistent of the S.T. heart attack subendocardial without vibe Q angina
unstable, angina of Prinzmetal Heart failure (35)
According to the clinical picture and electrocardiographic ischemic heart disease is classified into two large groups: painful ischemic heart disease and non-painful ischemic heart disease

HEART DISEASE PAINFUL ISCHEMIC

•Agina of recent start
•Agina of effort stable and of deterioration progressive
• Agina of repose: spontaneous, night, variant, postprandial
• Agina mixed
• Microangiopathic agina
• Agina pos heart attack

HEART DISEASE ISCHEMIC NO PAINFUL

•Death sudden
• Heart attack silent myocardium
•Insufficiency cardiac secondary to cardiomyopathy ischemic

•Disorder of the heart rate
•Disorder of the driving electric of the heart
•Disorder nonspecific of the repolarization ventricular (36) The angina according to the Spanish cardiology association is classified

AGINA STABLE AGINA UNSTABLE
• Agina of effort of recent beginning
•Agina progressive
•Agina of repose
• Prolonged agina
•Agina pos heart attack
• Agina variant (37)
The classification anatopathological of the heart attack of the myocardium according to The universal declaration of myocardial infarction 2007 is classified

BY HIS EVOLUTIONARY STATE

• Sharp
•Scarred
•Healing (37)

The classification functional of the heart disease according to New York Heart Association is classified

•Class I Is possible carry out the activity physical usual without that symptoms appear

•Class II He patient HE find asymptomatic in repose, but the activity physical usual produces symptoms
•Class III exist accented limitations in the activity physical and the Symptoms appear with less intense activities than usual

•Class IV He patient presents symptomatology in repose (38)
IN the research we worked with the forms of presentation of both acute and chronic ischemic heart disease, angina pectoris, heart failure and infarction

Ischemic heart disease can present as a chronic/stable disease (when there are stable atheromatous plaques, which usually manifest as stable stress angina, heart failure) or as an Acute Coronary Syndrome (ACS) (when an atheromatous plaque becomes unstable). , it gets complicated). (39)

Angina pectoris, Syndrome characterized by paroxysmal retrosternal pain characteristics that are triggered by exercise, emotions and other factors, rest and the use of nitroglycerin (40)

Etiology

Determining factors, narrowing of the coronary arteries in more than one 90%

Predisposing factors, arterial hypertension, habit of smoking, obesity, hyperlipidemia, diabetes mellitus, diet rich in saturated fats, stress and sedentary lifestyle (40)

Factors triggers Effort physical, emotions, cold, intercourse (40) Clinical Picture
It is characterized by pain, as a fundamental symptom that is characterized by being accompanied by psychic phenomena, such as It is fear and it is the feeling of eminent death. This location is retrosternal or precordial, oppressive compressive that appears after an effort that radiates to the left arm and is relieved with rest or with the administration of nitroglycerin (40).

Insufficiency Cardiac

Functional picture that reveals the inability of the heart to expel all the blood that arrives during diastole, making it impossible to maintain adequate cardiac output in relation to venous return and the needs of the body (41)

Classification

Right ventricular failure Failure ventricular left

Insufficiency cardiac global. Epidemiology
About 1% of the population over 40 years of age has heart failure. The prevalence of this disease doubles in each decade of age and is around 10% in those over 70 years of age. Cardiac incidence is a progressive and lethal disorder, even with adequate treatment.

Ethology

Hypertension Arterial
Valvulopathy mitral
Valvulopathy aortic diseases of the arteries coronary (42)

The coronary arteries are the arteries that supply the heart muscle, myocardium. They originate from the aortic sinuses of Valsalva. left and right valve. There are two: the right coronary artery and the left coronary artery. (43)

The right coronary artery emerges between the right atrial appendage and the origin of the pulmonary appendage, it enters the right atrioventricular sulcus and runs through it until it reaches the posterior interventricular sulcus, into which it is introduced and is then called the posterior interventricular artery. It is then divided into two main branches; the posterior descending artery and the right marginal artery (also called posterolateral). The right coronary artery primarily supplies the right ventricle and the lower region of the left ventricle The left coronary artery divides, almost immediately after its origin, into arterial falling former and artery circumflex. The artery falling former supplies the anterior and lateral aspects of the left ventricle in addition to the interventricular septum through its septal branches. The circumflex artery supplies the posterior aspect of the left ventricle. (44)

Dominance is defined by the artery from which the posterior descending branch originates, which in 85% is the right coronary artery (right dominance). In it The rest is the circumflex artery (left dominance), or there is co-dominance. (44)

Clinical Picture

Insufficiency ventricular left tachycardia
Dyspnoea

Displaced apex beat moves downward and to the left indicating an increase in the size of the left ventricle

Pulse alternating, sign of failed of the ventricle left
Cheyne Stoke breathing, breathing characterized by periods of hyperpnea and apnea as a result of cerebral ischemia

Insufficiency ventricular right
Painful hepatomegaly is the earliest objective symptom of insufficiency.

Oliguria, can decrease until 400 ml to the day

Peripheral edema, present in stages more advanced, painful hot edema and difficult to godet Engorgement venous jugular, increases in the position lying down and with liver compression. (Four. Five)

The Syndrome coronary sharp HE divide in:
- ACS with ST segment elevation (STEACS): Occurs when complicated atheromatous plaque produces complete obstruction of the coronary artery. It manifests on the electrocardiogram (ECG) with an elevation of the ST segment, and its treatment consists of acute reperfusion/opening of the vessel (either by means of drugs (fibrinolysis) or mechanically (primary angioplasty).

This treatment has to be realized in he minor time possible for avoid the myocardial necrosis. Less commonly, ST segment elevation may be due to coronary spasm. In this case, ST elevation is transient and usually resolves spontaneously or with nitrates. (46)

-ACS without ST segment elevation (NSTEACS): Occurs when complicated atheromatous plaque decreases flow through the affected vessel, but does not completely obstructs. Different changes are usually observed in the ECG of the elevation of the ST segment (a decrease in said segment is usually observed, but a negative T, isophasic, etc., may also appear). It can be managed in two ways, with an early aggressive strategy (which involves performing a cardiac catheterization in the first 72 hours, not immediately as in he case of the ACS either a strategy conservative (medical treatment, without performing, at least initially, cardiac catheterization). (46)

Definition universal of the heart attack sharp of myocardium (YO SOY) AMI can be recognized by clinical features, including ECG findings, elevation of biomarkers of myocardial necrosis, and imaging, or can be defined by pathologic criteria. (47)

In he past the WHO defined he YO SOY as symptoms ischemic, EKG compatible and elevation of myocardial necrosis enzymes. However, the development of very sensitive and specific markers of myocardial damage, and techniques of More sensitive imaging now allows the detection of very small amounts of myocardial necrosis. This requires a new definition. updated. The "third universal definition of myocardial infarction" is presented below. According to this, the term AMI should be used when there is evidence of myocardial necrosis in a clinical context of acute myocardial ischemia. Taking these conditions into account, any of the following criteria would imply the diagnosis of AMI: (48)

- Rise and fall of myocardial damage enzymes (preferably cardiac troponin) with at least one value above the 99th percentile of the upper reference limit with at least one of the following:

1. Symptoms of ischemia.
2. New either presumably new elevation significant of the segment

3. ST/ changes in the vibe T/new BRI.
4. Development of waves Q pathological in he ECG.
5.Evidence of loss of viable myocardium or new alteration of segmental motility evidenced by an imaging technique.

6. Identification of an intracoronary thrombus on angiography or autopsy - Death of cardiac origin with symptoms suggestive of myocardial ischemia and ischemic changes on the ECG or LBBB, when death occurred before cardiac biomarkers were obtained or before they had risen.

By other part, HE recognize the following definitions. (49)
Percutaneous coronary periprocedural AMI is arbitrarily defined as an elevation of cardiac troponin (>5 times the 99th percentile of normal) in patients with normal baseline values or an elevation greater than 20% if baseline values were altered. In addition,a) symptoms suggestive of ischemia either b) changes electrocardiographic new suggestive of ischemia either
c) changes angiographic compatible with a complication periprocedure either d) imaging demonstration of loss of viable myocardium or new alteration of segmental motility. (49)

He YO SOY associated to thrombosis of the stent HE define when HE detect by coronary angiography or autopsy in the setting of myocardial ischemia and with a rise and subsequent fall in markers of myocardial necrosis with at least one value above the 99th percentile. (49)

AMI associated with aorto-coronary bypass surgery is arbitrarily defined as an elevation in biomarkers of myocardial necrosis (>10 times the 99th percentile of normality) in patients with normal baseline values. Besides of a) new pathological Q waves, b) angiographic evidence of new occlusion of a bridge or a native vessel, or

c) imaging evidence of a loss of viable myocardium or a recent alteration of segmental contractility. - (49)

Any of the following criteria is diagnosis of YO SOY: (49)
- Waves Q pathological with either without symptoms in absence of causes No ischemic
- Imaging evidence of loss of viable myocardium that is thinned and not contracting adequately, in the absence of nonischemic causes

- Diagnosis anatomopathological of a YO SOY previous.

The incidence of ischemic heart disease, like most diseases, increases with age. Thus, the aging of the population is a determining factor in the increase in the importance of cardiovascular diseases, becoming one of the most important risk factors for suffering from chronic non-communicable diseases. (fifty)

At the threshold of the 21st century, Cuban society faces a demographic situation similar to that of developed countries, showing an increase in life expectancy that exceeds 75 years, at the same time it has a population of 60 years and further de1629184 population, it that It represents the 14 %of his population total, to the closing of 2015, so it is proposed that by 2020 this figure will reach 25% and will become the oldest country in Latin America (27)

Among cardiovascular diseases, coronary artery disease has a lot of weight in the elderly group. With the use of various diagnostic techniques to detect subclinical coronary artery disease, up to 22% of women and 33% of men between 65 and 70 years of age have been affected. This percentage increases considerably, up to 43% and 45% respectively, in people over 85 years of age. Likewise, old studies that have collected autopsy data show a prevalence of significant coronary heart disease of more than 50% in individuals over 70 years of age (exceeding 70% in male patients). In fact, although the population over 75 years does not reach to the 10% in the most developed countries, It represents almost 40% of patients hospitalized for acute coronary syndrome. Furthermore, the extent and severity of coronary artery disease in the elderly is greater compared to other age groups: the prevalence of three-vessel coronary artery disease, as well as left main coronary artery disease, increases with age. (51)

Regarding the type of ACS, non-ST elevation acute coronary syndrome (NSTEACS) is the most common clinical manifestation of ACS in the elderly. In the GRACE (Global Registry of Acute Coronary Events) registry, in which 14 countries participated, patients were divided into 5 age groups based on age, and it was observed that the proportion of patients with NSTEACS increased linearly with age. age, thus for those under 65 years of age the proportion was 30% and for those over 85 years of age it was 41%. On the contrary, coronary syndrome acute ST elevation syndrome (STEACS) was more common in younger patients (52)

This fact could be due to the higher prevalence of previous infarctions, multivessel disease, hypertension and ventricular hypertrophy that could produce global subendocardial ischemia and poor myocardial perfusion. (52)

Cardiovascular diseases are of multifactorial origin, and are related to lifestyle, especially tobacco consumption, unhealthy eating habits, physical inactivity and psychosocial stress.

According to the WHO, appropriate changes in lifestyle could prevent more than three quarters of mortality from cardiovascular diseases (53)

Among the non-modifiable cardiovascular risk factors, but which must be taken into account, are age, sex, race and family history of cardiovascular disease. premature (considered as factor risky he antecedent of the same in a first-degree relative in men before the age of 55 and in women before the age of 65). (54)

The distribution of cardiovascular risk factors is also different depending on age. The history of angina, cerebrovascular disease, myocardial infarction, heart failure, arterial hypertension and atrial fibrillation is more common in patients with Older. The only classic cardiovascular risk factor that is generally more prevalent in younger age groups is smoking. Thus, smoking is the only risk factor inversely associated with age. (55)

This may be explained either because smoking may not be an important CVRF in the elderly or because smokers may have lower survival after an ACS and therefore rarely reach adulthood. (56)

The clinical presentation of ACS is also different depending on age (more so in women greater); the elderly present with frequency symptoms atypical, so a high level of suspicion is necessary to avoid delays in treatment. (57)

Although chest pain continues to be the most common manifestation of AMI, dyspnea is a relatively common presentation in the elderly, perhaps due to the greater presence of systolic or diastolic dysfunction (57)

Furthermore, a high prevalence of silent ischemia has been described in the elderly, this is due to the fact that sensitivity to pain is reduced in the elderly, the greater presence of collateral circulation, an increase in the number of endorphin receptors and alterations of the autonomic nervous This leads to ischemic heart disease being frequently diagnosed by the manifestations of its complications more than those of the ischemic heart disease itself. (57)

Furthermore, the presence of basal alterations is more common in the elderly. in the ECG and atypical ECG, which makes it difficult to interpret and detect ischemia in stress tests, or the early diagnosis of ACS. (58)

Delay in seeking medical assistance is a common characteristic of heart attacks of the seniors. Maybe this HE explain by the high presence of atypical presentations, or by the presence of cognitive impairment that can mask the diagnosis of ACS. (58)

For years, knowledge about ischemic heart disease focused on men, due to the low participation of women in research work. In absolute figures, the female population with ischemic heart disease is larger (given the greater average female longevity), and the percentage of women is even higher in the oldest age group. (59)

The main differences lie in the presentation at a later age and in the presence of more comorbidity, such as diabetes mellitus, arterial hypertension and heart failure. Currently, it is already known that the clinical presentation of acute myocardial infarction is different in women. It has been observed that atypical presentation is more frequent, with less tendency to present chest pain and more back, head and jaw pain, abdominal discomfort, fatigue and dyspnea. (60)

Typical electrocardiographic signs are also less frequent in women, they tend to have less marked ST segment deviations. (61)

The effect of sex on the decisions of medical professionals has also been the subject of study. Women with chest pain are referred for catheterization less frequently than men, mainly when the diagnosis is uncertain. Differences in clinical presentation, in awareness about the probability of having a heart attack, and in the perception of medical personnel could determine a process of care different in the women, and especially in the elderly women. It would begin with a greater delay in diagnosis, followed by lower treatment intensity and higher mortality. In most studies of fatality after myocardial infarction, sex differences disappear or are attenuated when adjusting for delay in onset. diagnosis and performance of revascularization treatment (62)

The incidence of cardiac and non-cardiac complications increases progressively with age. Thus, the risk of atrial fibrillation, heart failure, recurrent ischemia or re-infarction is greater. The most frequent complication in the people of advanced age with SCA is the insufficiency cardiac, which can appear in up to 50% of patients. It is well known that mortality is higher in patients who develop heart failure after a heart attack than in those who do not. (63)

Such a high incidence of heart failure is not caused by a higher infarct size, but is due to the different response of the senile left ventricle to ischemia. The left ventricle is characterized by presenting with he aging a dysfunction diastolic progressive. The ischemia Myocardial dysfunction produces a slowdown in ventricular relaxation and an increase in end-diastolic pressure of the left ventricle. Therefore, the physiological alterations of aging aggravate the pathological consequences of heart attack and translate into a high incidence of pulmonary edema, which is not always a consequence of the systolic dysfunction produced by the infarction. (64)

The first cause of Death in heart attack is cardiogenic shock, whose incidence in the population old woman is approximately of the twenty%. Besides, with the age No It only increases the incidence of shock but also its lethality. cardiogenic shock can occur by dysfunction of anyone of the ventricles or both. Cardiogenic shock due to left ventricular dysfunction is much more common in anterior infarctions and in very extensive infarctions. Cardiogenic shock due to right ventricular dysfunction is almost exclusive to infarcts of the inferior aspect and generally due to occlusion of the right coronary artery at a proximal level. This complication increases exponentially with age, affecting up to 40% of octogenarians with lower AMI and right ventricular involvement. (65)

On the other hand, rhythm disorders are very common in the acute phase of a heart attack in the elderly. Atrial fibrillation is particularly common. Atrioventricular block is also more common and its appearance in the acute phase is associated with a worse short-term prognosis. The incidence of primary ventricular fibrillation, unlike other rhythm disorders, and mechanical complications are the second most common cause of death. in STEACS. There are basically three: free wall rupture, ventricular septal defect (VSD) and papillary muscle rupture. Its incidence increases progressively with age. The most frequent among mechanical complications of heart attack is the rip of wall free, further associated to anterior and lateral infarcts. Papillary muscle tears are more common in inferior infarcts. All of them are almost exclusive to ST elevation infarctions. Among the elderly we observed a higher incidence of mechanical complications in women, non-smokers, dyslipidemic patients and those without a history of angina prior to the infarction. (66)

In black patients the incidence of ischemic heart disease is much higher. This is because they are more predisposed to suffering from hypertension, which favors artery sclerosis. It is estimated that on average men have 6mmHg higher resting systolic pressure than their white counterparts, and that women have up to 17mmHg, which is the population group of higher risk. Black individuals have greater survival after a heart attack than white individuals. Epidemiological studies have shown that both black and Asian people have a tendency to suffer from the disease. insulin resistance syndrome, in which insulin stops performing its function and favors the appearance of abdominal obesity and dyslipidemia, a factor that would also explain (25)

In adult patients with AMI, the genetic component has been estimated to contribute between 20-40%. Multiple studies show that the risk in siblings of patients with manifestations of ischemic heart disease is 25 times greater than in control individuals. There are several genetic alterations that appear in various families that could explain the predisposition to suffer AMI, among these we find the association between the 4G/5G polymorphism in the plasminogen activator inhibitor gene. (67)

A risk factor, is an element or a measurable characteristic that has a causal relationship with the development of a disease, hence its importance in its identification and his assessment. The ID and assessment of the factors of cardiovascular risk, allows stratifying patients in risk groups and implement pharmacological and non-pharmacological intervention measures that contribute to risk reduction or control. (68) Factors of risk modifiable There is clear evidence of the adverse effect of tobacco on health, with smoking being responsible for approximately 50% of preventable deaths. Half of these deaths are due to cardiovascular disease (69). The risk of heart attack is much higher among smokers than among non-smokers, and the rate of sudden death is increased more than 10 times in men and more than 5 times in women who smoke. (70). The effect of tobacco is related to the amount of tobacco consumed and the duration of the smoking habit. (70)

Smoking is considered the main risk factor in heart attack patients. In developed countries, it reaches the level of being the main cause of early morbidity and mortality, being responsible for more than half of preventable mortality, especially cardiovascular mortality. By 2025, it is estimated that 10 billion deaths related to tobacco consumption will occur annually because it accelerates atherogenesis, increases the oxidation of LDL-cholesterol and decreases HDL-cholesterol, and prevents dependent vasodilation of the coronary arteries. of the endothelium, increases platelet aggregation and increases the prevalence of coronary spasm.(71)

Diabetes mellitus is a major risk factor for coronary heart disease and ictus. Various prospective studies have shown that type 2 diabetes has double the risk of coronary heart disease and stroke, increasing by 2 to 4 times the mortality from these diseases (Fox, 2007). So much so, that it has been considered that the risk of cardiovascular disease in subjects with type 2 diabetes is similar to that of patients with a previous myocardial infarction. HE ha observed that levels elevated of hemoglobin glycosylated, Even in the range of values currently considered normal, they increase cardiovascular risk. (72)

The pathophysiology of vascular disease in Diabetes Mellitus involves abnormalities of endothelial function, smooth muscle cells, and skin function. Hyperglycemia, excess free fatty acids and insulin resistance favor a complex traffic of molecular signals that alter the function and even the structure of the vascular wall, through 3 main mechanisms: oxidative stress, activation of protein kinase C (PKC) and stimulation of receptors for advanced glycation products (RAGE). This complex process converges towards vasoconstriction due to lower availability of nitric oxide (NO), release of vasoactive agents such as endothelin (ET) and angiotensin II (AII), inflammatory mediators due to the activation of nuclear factor kappa beta (NF-K B) and a prothrombotic environment due to increased release of tissue factor (TF) and PAI. Vasoconstriction, inflammation and thrombosis are the basic ingredients for the development of atherothrombotic disease, which can lead to acute myocardial infarction. (72)

With respect to dyslipidemia, the association between cholesterol levels and cardiovascular disease is also influenced by the presence of other cardiovascular risk factors associated with dyslipidemia. The presence of diabetes or high levels of triglycerides, or low levels of HDL cholesterol aggravates the effects of total cholesterol, even if its levels are only slightly elevated. This reason is fundamental for the global estimation of cardiovascular risk. The presence of triglyceride levels > 1.7 mmol/l (150 mg/dl) is one of the criteria used in the definition of metabolic syndrome. (73) A meta-analysis by John Hokanson confirms triglycerides as an independent risk factor for coronary heart disease. For every 1 mmol/L increase in them the risk of coronary heart disease increased 37% in women and 14% in men. Several factors explain the effect of hypertriglyceridemia as a risk factor for coronary heart disease, among them we can mention that hypertriglyceridemia enables the appearance of LDL plus dense and small and therefore more atherogenic, there is also a decrease of HDL, which is what carries out reverse transport, which explains, in part, the coronary risk of this disorder (73).

Regarding high blood pressure (HTN), a few decades ago it was observed that its treatment resulted in a reduction in those clinical complications directly related to the moderate or severe elevation of blood pressure in proportion to the decrease in blood pressure. the blood pressure obtained with treatment. In the last years HE ha observed as he Treatment of mild HTN also results in a reduction in coronary morbidity and mortality. (74)

Hypertension represents greater resistance for the heart, which responds by increasing its muscle mass (left ventricular hypertrophy) to cope with this overstrain. This increase in muscle mass ends up being harmful because it is not accompanied by an equivalent increase in blood flow and can cause coronary insufficiency and angina pectoris. In addition, the heart muscle becomes more irritable and more arrhythmias occur. (75)

In patients who have already had a cardiovascular problem, hypertension can intensify the damage. High blood pressure leads to arteriosclerosis (accumulation of cholesterol in the arteries) and phenomena of thrombosis (can cause myocardial infarction or cerebral infarction). At worst In most cases, hypertension can soften the walls of the aorta and cause it to dilate (aneurysm) or rupture, which inevitably leads to death. (76)

High blood pressure is associated with a higher rate of asymptomatic heart attacks and a higher rate of mortality and complications during the acute phase of the heart attack. Five-year survival is almost 30% higher in normotensive subjects. In patients over 60 years of age, reducing systolic blood pressure below 160 reduces overall mortality, as well as cardiovascular mortality (77).

Several physiological changes occur in the elderly, such as a decrease in metabolism. basal, redistribution of the composition bodily, alterations in he functioning of the digestive system, modification in sensory perception, in chewing capacity, decreased sensitivity to thirst, loss of body mass, increased frequency and severity of diseases non-communicable chronic diseases and side effects of drugs that directly and indirectly affect nutritional status.(78)

However, of all the modifications, andrometric measurements are the most affected, highlighting body mass and height, which is why it is considered normal for the person. elderly a body mass index of 22 to 27 kg square meters, subjects with a height less than 1.50m should be considered with a cut-off point greater than 25 kg square meters. (90) Currently, there is great evidence that obesity in older adults increases cardiometabolic risk.

Obesity determines various risks in the biological, psychological and social sphere. Biological risks manifest themselves in the short, medium and long term through different diseases. , the risk of sudden death it's three times elderly. The obesity reduces Life expectancy between 5 and 8 years. (79) In cardiovascular diseases, it has been a matter of controversy whether obesity alone is an independent risk factor for atherosclerotic coronary heart disease or exerts its influence as a conditioning element of other factors, especially high blood pressure, diabetes, and dyslipidemia. He Framinglam study showed that for every 10% weight increase, blood pressure increases 65mmHg, plasma cholesterol 12mg. Vega demonstrated in 1947, 1956, that in the obesity of predominance thoracoabdominal there was elderly frequency of intolerance to the glucose, dyslipidemia, and hypertension, with an increased cardiovascular risk (79)

DESIGN METHODOLOGICAL

A case-control analytical study was carried out, where we worked with the total of 34 patients, older adults, diagnosed with ischemic heart disease, from the Family Medical Office 8, belonging to the Manacas Teaching Polyclinic, Santo Domingo municipality, province of Villa Clara, during the period from September 2019 to December 2021, and was paired with a control group. Mating was carried out 1:1, homogenizing by sex.

Criteria of Inclusion, cases:

- They reside in the area served by the Family Medical Office 8 belonging to the Manacas Teaching Polyclinic
- Patients with diagnosis of heart disease corroborated with the internal medicine specialist with dispensing and monitoring of your disease
- That they accepted participate in he study. (Exhibit 1) Exclusion criteria, cases:
- Refusal to participate in the study.

Criteria of Inclusion, controls:

- Patients who, after medical evaluation, do not present a diagnosis of cardiovascular involvement and who decide through their consent to be part of the study

Criteria of exclusion, controls:

- Patients chosen to belong to the control group who did not agree to participate in the study.

Data collection method: an interview was conducted where age, sex, smoking habit, family history of ischemic heart disease were explored in both groups (Annex 2), individual medical records were studied, using a documentary review guide. , (Annex 3)

Prosecution of the information:

All information was stored in a database made up of the statistical package SPSS vs. 15 for Windows, where all the processing took place .Absolute and relative frequency distributions expressed in number were used. and by hundred, HE calculation the Reason of Advantage (OR), according to the values OR=1 is not a risk factor, OR>1 is a risk factor, OR<1 is a protective factor Finally, the results were expressed in statistical tables for better interpretation.

Operationalization of Variables:

AGE: HE express in years compliments in he moment of the diagnosis for he cluster of the cases their categories were:

- **65 to 70 years.**
- **Elderly 70 years old.**

SEX consisted in he sex biological with that HE is born and HE classified in:

- **male.**
- **female.**

COLOR OF THE SKIN here HE consider two categories

- **White**
- **Not white**

GUY OF HEART DISEASE : According to the shape of presentation of the same, HE they took

three categories:

- **Angina**
- **myocardial infarction**
- **Insufficiency cardiac**

FACTORS OF RISK OF HEART DISEASE : HE they considered for he study

factors established by the literature and HE picked up the information of each one according to his presence or not

- **Smoking habit** : the person reports having smoked always or at some time in their life or at least 5 years before the diagnosis of heart disease.
- **APP diabetes:** here HE they considered the patients with diagnosis of Diabetes mellitus prior to ischemic heart disease.

- **APP of hypertension arterial** : here HE they considered the patients with a diagnosis of arterial hypertension prior to ischemic heart disease
- **Dyslipidemia** here HE they considered the patients with diagnosis of dyslipidemia prior to ischemic heart disease
- **Obesity** here HE they considered the patients with diagnosis of obesity prior to ischemic heart disease

Ethics of the investigation

The voluntariness of those involved in the study was taken into account at all times. Before beginning the data collection, an informed consent document was applied which explains that the study results will only be for research purposes, and all the rights that assist you as a patient will be respected, as well as the different procedures and techniques that will be carried out. during the investigation. Appendix 1.

RESULTS

- Of the 3. 4 Adults greater from the office 8 diagnosed with ischemic heart disease in the period 2019-2020, table 1, 21 for 61.7% belonged to the male sex and 79.5% were between ages above 70 years. 50% of the cases in study coincided in be male over 70 years old

- In the distribution of older adults with ischemic heart disease in office 8, Manacas health area according to skin color, table 2, of a total of 34 patients with ischemic heart disease, 25 are white. that represented a 73.52%, 9 No white it that represented a 26.47%,

of the total.

- The distribution of cases according to type of heart disease showed that 47.05% presented angina, followed by 32.35% with heart failure and in 7 patients, which represented 20.58%, coronary syndrome was found. Sharp. Table 3
- Table 4 shows the distribution of cases and controls with respect to the presence of first-degree family pathological history of ischemic heart disease in the older adult of CMF8 belonging to

to the health area of the Manacas polyclinic where it was observed that in 29 cases, which represented 85.29%, a family pathological history was found. of 1st line and only in he 52.94% of the controls HE confirmed the presence of this risk factor. The statistical analysis showed that the antecedent pathological familiar of heart disease ischemic in familiar of first line in this population constitutes a risk factor for developing the entity under study and the probability of developing ischemic heart disease in patients with background family pathological history of heart disease in the first line is 5 times more than those who do not have this family pathological history

- When distributing patients according to habit of smoking table 5 was observed that 28 cases that represented 82.35% are smokers, and only in he

The presence of smoking was confirmed in 67.64% of the controls. The statistical analysis showed that smoking in this population constitutes a risk factor for developing the entity under study and the probability of developing ischemic heart disease in smoking patients is 2.23 times more likely than those who are not smokers.

- Table 6 shows the distribution of the groups with respect to the presence of a personal pathological history of diabetes mellitus. in the older adult of CMF8 belonging to the health area of the Manacas polyclinic where HE noticed that in 18 cases that represented a 52.94%. HE

found a personal pathological history of diabetes mellitus and only 8.82% of the controls found the presence of this risk factor. The statistical analysis showed that the pathological history diabetes mellitus in this population constitutes a risk factor for developing the entity under study and the probability of developing a heart disease ischemic in patients with background pathological individuals of diabetes mellitus are 12 times more likely than those that do not have this background.

- When we analyze he behavior of the hypertension arterial in both groups, table 7, it was observed that in 33 cases, which represented 97.05%, a personal pathological history of arterial hypertension was found, and only in 58.82%of controls HE confirmed the presence of this factor of risk. The statistical analysis showed that the pathological history Personal hypertension in this population constitutes a risk factor for developing the entity under study and the probability of developing ischemic heart disease in patients with a personal pathological history of arterial hypertension is 23 times more likely than those who do not have a personal pathological history of hypertension. arterial
- In the distribution of patients according to the presence of dyslipidemia in both study groups, table 8, it was observed that in 28 cases which represented 82.35% had a personal pathological history of dyslipidemia and only in 23.52%of controls HE confirmed the presence of this risk factor for developing the entity under study and the probability of developing ischemic heart disease in patients with a personal pathological history of dyslipidemia is 15 times more likely than those who do not have a personal pathological history of dyslipidemia

- In the comparison of both groups according to personal pathological history of obesity, Table 9 showed that in 32 cases, which represented 94.11%, a personal pathological history of obesity was found and only in 70.58% of controls was the presence of this risk factor found. to develop the entity under study and the probability of developing a heart disease ischemic in patients with background personal pathological history of obesity is 6 times more likely than those who do not have a personal pathological history of obesity.

DISCUSSION OF THE RESULTS

The increase in life expectancy that has occurred in recent decades, related to the improvement in the quality of life and fundamentally with advances in medicine, has as a consequence an increase in the aging of the population. Individuals are reaching ages that were unthinkable in previous times, and the number of octogenarians has increased (80)As human beings are not capable of surviving many chronic diseases, when one suffers from a condition that inexorably leads to Death, quality of life and the risk of suffering from them become the main concern of healthcare physicians and researchers. Worthily preventing the appearance, timely diagnosis and reducing the complications of these diseases as much as possible is the objective in diseases incurable. Knowledge of those factors, modifiable or not, that influence the appearance, is a critical aspect to achieve this objective. (80)

The heart disease ischemic in he adult elderly ha been studied and according to the literature regarding the condition, according to sex and age, we find differences and similarities in the studies carried out in different regions, and also in the incidence by sex in relation to age, Thus, the author Gonzales Ramírez in a study carried out in Colombia states that each year, the incidence rates of acute myocardial infarction ranged between 135-210 new cases per year per year. each 100,000 men and between 29-61 by each 100,000 women between 25 and 74 years. AND Yeah the incidence HE measured in population elderly of 69 years the rates HE would elevate to 2,371 in men and 1,493 in women, this makes this pathology the main cause of death in both men and women, the maximum frequency age is over 65, with the male sex predominating over the female sex (81) . On the other hand, in studies carried out by Steptoe and his group, they established the differences that occur in the cardiovascular response (blood pressure, heart rate, baroreceptor reflex) and in the endocrine response to different stressful tasks. The results obtained suggest that, although the cardiovascular response is more prominent in young men than in adults, in the latter there is an inhibition of the baroreceptor reflex. This implies a readjustment to higher blood pressure levels, which would indicate the existence of a structural adaptation determined by age. These same studies also show manifest that cardiovascular reactivity is much greater in males than in females (82), Antonio Álvarez in one of his studies suggests that advanced age is associated with a high risk of suffering from ischemic heart disease; With age, sympathetic activity increases and the sensitivity of the baroreceptors and the regulatory response capacity of the systems decrease, systolic blood pressure and all markers of atherosclerosis and arterial stiffness and pulse pressure, among other metabolic, involutional and apoptotic effects, thus the older you are, the greater the chances of suffering from associated diseases (83). De Backer also considers the male gender as an important risk factor for the development of acute myocardial infarction (84). Velázquez – Monroy and Avezum report a predominance of the male sex for this disease. Our results fully agree with those indicated by these authors since in the population of clinic 8, ischemic heart disease predominated in men over 70 years of age, only a third of the study population belonged to the female sex, so we disagree with what was published by Dr. Liliam Gretel Cisneros Sánchez, in an article published in Revista Cubana de Medicina General Integral 2013, where A predominance of cases with ischemic heart disease is demonstrated in the female sex, represented by 53.8% of the selected sample.Regarding the most frequent age for the development of heart disease in the different bibliographies, we find that Bertomeu cites a higher prevalence of coronary heart disease in patients aged greater than or equal to 65 years (68.3%) and reports an OR 2.5 higher in the old man. Gonzales Ramírez already indicates a greater probability over 69 years of age (81), authors with whom we agree since in our population three quarters are over 70 years of age. Skin color is a known cardiovascular risk factor. Dr. Orestes Días Castro on the characterization of vascular risk factors in adult patients in the municipality of Ranchuelo Villa Clara, Cuba suggests that the white race predominated with 82.7% in patients with heart disease ischemic (86), on the other hand, Dr. Yaisel Alfonso Alfonso, in a study on the characterization of risk factors in patients with ischemic heart disease, suggests that the white race predominated in patients with a personal pathological history of heart disease (87). Our research coincides with the aforementioned studies, these statistics differ from what was proposed by The Society Spanish of cardiology. (88) that points out that in the individuals of race black the incidence of ischemic heart disease is higher. We agree with Dr. Castro Gutiérrez in a study on ischemic heart disease and complications, which states that ischemic heart disease most frequently affected white patients, followed by black patients, related to the demographic distribution and ethnicity of the Cuban population. (89)

According to the distribution of patients by type of heart disease, it was observed that angina is more frequent in older adults belonging to office 8 from the town of Manaca. Coinciding with a similar study carried out in the municipality of Sagua la Grande, Villa Clara Cuba, where angina prevailed as the main form of clinical presentation of ischemic heart disease (86). Besides in a study by Dr. Orestes Días Castro on the characterization of vascular risk factors in adult patients in the municipality of Ranchuelo Villa Clara, Cuba states that of the total number of patients studied with ischemic heart disease, those who further prevalent were the angina of chest and he heart attack sharp of myocardial infarction (87) We agree with the studies presented above, but not completely because in our research myocardial infarction was the least frequency.The background in relatives of first degree of heart disease HE they mention in literature as one of the determinants of coronary risk, studies suggest that Most of the known genetic alterations related to atherosclerosis affect lipoprotein metabolism (90).

Families in which a member has suffered a cardiovascular event are considered as of high risk already that the genetics either the habits bit healthy are transmitted to offspring (90). Leander suggests in his study carried out in Stockholm that family members who share genes, as well as the environment, habits and lifestyle can be associated with a lower or higher risk of cardiovascular diseases (91).

In these aspects our research fully agrees because We confirmed that the majority of patients had a pathological history in first-degree relatives with heart disease.

In a study carried out in 2016 by Dr. Radka Ivanova, it was evident that 85% of patients with ischemic heart disease had a family history. of disease coronary with presentation clinic early before of the
55 years for men and 65 years for women of these (92) Our research agrees with what was proposed by this doctor since there was a great predominance of older adult patients with heart disease with a family history of the disease

It is estimated that between 20 and 30% of all deaths from coronary heart disease in the United States are attributable to tobacco use and the risk is strongly dose related, a acute coronary disease anticipates approximately 10 years in smokers in relation to non-smokers. By quitting tobacco, the risk of morbidity and mortality decreases cardiovascular. The risk increases directly with the number of cigarettes smoked per day (92), coinciding with the results of various authors such as Kliver M who propose that smoking is one of the major risk factors for the disease cardiovascular, the nicotine favors he development of the cardiovascular disease through its action on the autonomic nervous system with the release of catecholamines, increased platelet aggregation, lipid alterations and endothelial dysfunction(93)

Dr. Resano Berrio suggests that the risk of myocardial infarction is much higher among smokers than among non-smokers, and the risk of sudden death is increased more than 10 times in men and more than 5 times in women who smoke. . The effect of tobacco is related to the amount of tobacco consumed and with the duration of the smoking habit. (94)

In a study carried out in 2016 by Dr. Julio Cesar Calero Fierro, it is evident that 58.18% of older adults who died from ischemic heart disease HE attributed to the smoking. (69) Our investigation it matches with what was proposed by this doctor since there was a great predominance of smoking patients with a diagnosis of the disease, the statistical results show the probability of developing ischemic heart disease in patients with smoking habits and the appearance of the disease.

In he study of the Dr. Marvin José Vanegas Vanegas poses that the reduction of coronary risk after stopping smoking, it is evident after a year. Smoking alone increases the risk of coronary heart disease by two times (13); very similar results in terms of probability were obtained in the present study.

The Framingham study found an increase in cardiovascular mortality of 18% in men and 36% in women who consumed more than 3 to 10 cigarettes a day (70). In a study carried out in 2017 by Dr. Jaromir Pastora Benavides, it is evident that 40.6% of older adults who died from ischemic heart disease It was attributed to smoking increasing the risk of heart disease in the elderly by 3.4 (71). Our study coincides with this author, although the probabilities identified in the population of older adults from medical office 8 in the town of Manaca were slightly lower than those published by the author. Our research coincides with previous ones since smoking behaved as a predisposing factor for the development of ischemic heart disease.

The pathophysiology of vascular disease in Diabetes Mellitus involves abnormalities of endothelial function, smooth muscle cells, and platelet function. Hyperglycemia, excess free fatty acids and insulin resistance favor a complex traffic of molecular signals. that alter the function and even the structure of the vascular wall, through 3 main mechanisms: oxidative stress, activation of protein kinase C (PKC) and stimulation of receptors for advanced glycation products (RAGE). This complex process converges towards vasoconstriction due to lower availability of nitric oxide (NO), release of vasoactive agents such as endothelin (ET) and angiotensin II (AII), inflammatory mediators due to the activation of nuclear factor kappa beta (NF-K B) and a prothrombotic environment due to increased release of factor tissue (FT) and PAI. The vasoconstriction, inflammation and Thrombosis are the basic ingredients for the development of atherothrombotic disease, which can lead to acute myocardial infarction (72).

A history of diabetes mellitus is mentioned in the literature as a factor that influences the appearance of ischemic heart disease; studies suggest its presence as a significant increase in the risk of suffering from cardiovascular diseases, since it leads to an increase in blood levels. of atherosclerosis, and the early appearance of lesions causing 70% of deaths in patients with diabetes, being its presence in the general population of 6% and gradually increasing as the population ages. In this aspect, our research fully agrees since we confirmed that more than half of the cases had a personal pathological history. of diabetes mellitus (72)

Dr. Roka Ivanova Giorgeva states that in individuals with glucose intolerance there is a one- to two-fold increased risk of developing macrovascular disease (95). In our population, the probability of developing heart disease in patients with diabetes mellitus was much higher. to the one found by this author

In the study Dr. (Evans, 2002) suggests that high levels of glycosylated hemoglobin, even in the range of values currently considered normal, increase cardiovascular risk (26)

In a publication made in Argentina in 2015 by Dr. Cristina Del Bosque Martin Teacher headline of medicine internal poses that the diabetes mellitus is a major risk factor for coronary heart disease, which has double the risk in the incidence of coronary heart disease, increasing of 2 to 4 times the mortality from these diseases. So much so, that it has been considered that the risk of cardiovascular disease in subjects with type 2 diabetes is similar to that of patients with a previous myocardial infarction (29). Our results also exceed the probabilities found in Dr. Cristina's study population. The personal history of diabetes mellitus in older adults in office 8 of the Manacas health area was ranked as the third risk factor in probability for the development of ischemic heart disease.

The incidence of arterial hypertension in older adults is closely related to ischemic heart disease; in fact, it is considered that for every increase of 20 mmHg in systolic blood pressure (SBP) or 10 mmHg in diastolic blood pressure (DBP), the risk is doubled. risk of acute myocardial infarction, throughout the range from 115/75 to 185/115 mmHg, estimating that there is a continuous, consistent relationship and independent of other factors, such as a dose-response association. In a study carried out by the World Health Organization, an estimated 8 to 18% suffer from high blood pressure, and indicates that a 2mmHg decrease in blood pressure Average arterial pressure reduces deaths caused by cardiovascular diseases by around 4%. (75)

In a study carried out by the American Society of Hypertension, according to Dr. Arocha HE considers that the pressure arterial has to be conceptualized as a continuous risk factor in older adults in the context of cardiovascular risk (77)

In a study carried out by Dtr Lewinton on the behavior in age groups related to blood pressure and vascular mortality, it is considered that between the ages 40 and 49 years and 80 and 89 years HE associate the double of the death rate from ischemic heart disease, increasing the absolute risk (75)

In a case-control analytical study carried out by the author Maikel Santos M, it is noted that 87.3% of hypertensive patients, with OR = 3.610 (95% CI: 1.073- 21.843), p = 0.044, were statistically significant with the in-hospital mortality due to AMI in old age (24)

Our research coincides with the aforementioned studies, resulting in a very high probability according to the OR values. Which placed it as the factor that most likely contributed to coronary heart disease in older adults in clinic 8 of Manacas in the study period.

With high cholesterol levels, according to the literature regarding heart disease in older adults, we find similarities in the studies carried out in different regions, as well in a study carried out Multiple Risk Factors Interventional Trial". A significant relationship is proposed between cholesterol levels above 250 mg/dl and the incidence of IHD. Furthermore, they noted that differences in serum cholesterol between different populations were largely due to dietary saturated fat intake (96). The Multiple Study risk Factors Interventional Trial poses that the relationship between the levels plasmatic of cholesterol and he risk of IC was gradual, without a threshold specific (9). On the other hand, the Framingham study suggests a clear relationship between the increase in total cholesterol and/or LDL cholesterol and the subsequent risk of developing IC. There is also an inverse relationship between HDL cholesterol levels and the risk of heart disease (97). In a study carried out by Dr. Altamirano, a specialist in internal medicine in 2016, a probability of 1.4 times further of Heart attack of myocardium in patients dyslipidemic

(98). In a publication made in Mexico in 2016 by Dr. Jaromir Ramón Pastora Benavides. Internal Medicine Resident suggests that presenting some type of Dyslipidemia increases the risk of Acute Coronary Syndrome to almost 10 times more. (99) These results are lower than the probability found in our study population. We agree that lipid disorders promote coronary heart disease, dyslipidemia was ranked as the second risk factor with the highest probability of developing ischemic heart disease in older adults of CMF 8 during 2019 and 2020.

Obesity is a known cardiovascular risk factor. Studies carried out in Western countries have shown a relationship between obesity and cardiovascular mortality. In a study carried out by ACS, the American Cancer Society shows that each increase of 1 in body mass index corresponds to an increase of 1.1 in the relative risk of cardiovascular death in men aged 65 to 74 years and in women of this age it is 1.03. (100) In a study by Dr. Jaromir Ramón Pastora Benavides. Internal Medicine Resident about he behavior of the factors of risk associates to syndrome acute coronary suggests that being overweight increases cardiovascular risk twice as much (99)

In a study by Dr. KATHERIN LISBETH VILCHEZ CABRER on the behavior of risk factors associated with acute coronary syndrome, it suggests that obesity and early coronary disease in a first-degree relative increase the prevalence of suffer a event coronary in 2.4 times and
1.41 times consecutively (101), on the other hand, in a study by (American Association, it is proposed that an increase in abdominal and/or visceral fat is related to biochemical and clinical disorders that can increase cardiovascular risk (100)

Our research coincides with the aforementioned studies by pointing out obesity as a predisposing factor that occupied the most importance in the sample. fourth place in order of priority within other factors studied

CONCLUSIONS

In the 2019-2020 stage, ischemic heart disease in older adults in office 8 of the Manacas area predominates in male patients and increases directly proportional to age. Angina is the most common. All the factors studied behaved as predisposing factors for the development of heart disease, including high blood pressure, dyslipidemia and diabetes mellitus, in that order.

RECOMMENDATIONS

Recommend based on identified factors develop interventions that allow the control and reduction of them to avoid injuries.Ischemic heart disease in older adults

REFERENCES BIBLIOGRAPHICAL

1. Scanned Barbossa Brief history from the heart and of the cardiological knowledge. Madrid, 2016

2. Bazzino EITHER Third definition universal of heart attack of myocardium Uruguay 2018

3. Ruiz AND Factors of risk cardiovascular in greater of 80 years available at: https:/ /www.scielo . org.pe/scielo

4. Rail I, Medina F . Strategies of reperfusion used in patients with acute coronary syndrome without ST segment elevation. ,Madrit 2019

5. Organization world of the Health, Diseases Cardiovascular 2017 [website]. [cited Dec 18, 2017]. Available at: http://www.who.int/es/newsroom/fact-sheet/detail /cardiovascular - diseases

6. Bonow R, Mann D, Zips D, Treaty of Cardiology 2 day Edition 2016, chapter 50

7. Aje TO, Miller M. Cardiovascular disease: a global problem extending into the developing world. World J Cardiol 2016

8. Vanegas V. Marvin. Factors associates acute myocardial infarction in patients admitted in he hospital Anthony Lenin Fonseca during he 2015. Thesis for obtain he Qualification of Specialist in Emergency. 2016, Nicaragua.

9. Royo-Bordonada M, Cupboard Q, Wolves Bejarano J, Botet J, Villar Álvarez F, Elosua R. Spanish adaptation of the 2016 European guides on prevention of disease cardiovascular in the practice clinic. Rev. Esp Public Health [internet].2016 . Available at http://www.msc.es/resp. http://www.ceipc.inf .

10. Melo-Barbosa EITHER. Disease cardiovascular: beliefs and practices in adherence to treatment. Rev Cienc. City [internet]. Available at http://www.dx.doi.org/10.22463/1794831.1410. pdf 12. Archury-Beltran L. Validity and reliability of the questionnaire for measure I

11. Brant I, Moraes D, Ribeiro TO. Health global and disease cardiovascular. Rev Uruguay Cardiol [Internet]. 2015 [consultation 06 of September 2018]; Available at http://www.scielo.edu.uy > scielo.pdf

12. González Juanatey J. new therapeutic approach for secondary prevention of the risk cardiovascular. Rev Esp Cardiol [Internet]. 2017 Available in http://www.scielo.edu.uy > scielo.pdf

13. Texas heart Institute. Factors of risk cardiovascular. 2018. [Internet]. Available in: https://www.texasheart.org/hearthealth/heart- information-

center/topics/cardiovascular-risk-factors/

14. Reis E, Takao C, Zimmer A, Batista V, De Lima J, Leite A. Association of cardiovascular risk factors with the different presentations of the syndrome coronary sharp. Rev Latin-American of Enfermagem. [Online]. 2019. [], Vol 22 N°04. Available at http://www.scielo.br/scielo.php?pid=S010411692014000400538&script =sci_arttext&tlng=e
15. Dr. Albert Caccavo, He heart attack sharp of myocardium, a problem of public health; Rev. argent. cardiol. vol.78 no. Ecuador May/Jun. 2016

16. Car TO., Bastiaenen R., Kaski J.C. Disease cardiovascular in the old man: comment.Rev Esp Cardiol. 2016

17. Prieto Dominguez T ,Twelve Rodriguez V, serra Valdez MA .Factors `predictors of mortality in heart attack sharp of myocardium. Rev Finlay [internet].2017 available http://scielo.sld.cu/.php/scrip/
18. Population and development study center. The aging of the Cuban Population and its territories [internet]. Havana National office of Statistics,2009 [aforementioned 14 January 2016].Available at http://www . One.cu.sld.cu/. publications/cepede/ aging /aging 2009. ´pdf
19. Rocabruno Mederos JC.Treaty of gerantology and geriatrics clinic. Havana Scientific and Technical 2016

20. Landrave O Gómez. Epidemiological transition and chronic diseases No transmissible in the Americas and in Cuba, he program of Cuban intervention. Surveillance technical report 2016
21. Ministry of Health Public. Yearbook Statistical of Health 2020 [Internet]. Havana : Address National of Records Doctors and Health Statistics; Apr 2020 [cited Jan 10, 2020]. Available at http://files.sld.cu/dne/files/2020/04/anuario_2020.pdf

22. Santos R, Naples M. Behavior of the heart attack sharp of myocardium in older adults treated at the XX Anniversary Polyclinic. CorSalud 2016

23. Office National of Statistics and Information. Yearbook Statistical 2019. town clear
24. Santos M, Lanas, f., Toro, V., Cortes, R., Sánchez, A. (2008). Interheart, a Study of cases and controls about factors of risk of Heart attack of Myocardium in the World and Latin America. Reflection on an original article. Magazine of the students of the Industrial University of Santander Medicas UIS. Available at: http://www.medicasuis.org/anteriores/volumen21.3/5.pdf

25. Gomez Sanchez, G., Castellanos olive groves, TO. (2015). Factors of Cardiovascular Risk in the Geriatric Patient: Primary and Secondary Prevention. Identification of Perioperative Risk. Vol. 28 (1), 189-196 Available at: http://web.a.ebscohost.com/ehost/pdfviewer/pdfviewer?sid=b359edfd- 8d2d-4727-a264-64e271268972%40sessionmgr4008&vid=5&hid=410

26. Velez C, Gil I, Avila C, Lopez TO. Factors of risk cardiovascular and associated variables in people aged 20 to 79 years in Manizales, Colombia. University and Health. 2015

27. Ramiro Rodriguez M. He problem of the heart disease ischemic in Cuba Available at http://bvs.sld.cu/revistas/res/vol14

28. Aje TO, Miller M. Cardiovascular disease: a global problem extending into the developing world. World J Cardiol 2018;

29. Allender S, Scarborough P, Peto V, Rayner M, Leal J, Luengo-Fernandez R, et al. European Cardiovascular Disease Statistics 2017 Edition. European Heart Network; 2017;

30. Baena Ten J.M., of the Val Garcia J.L., Thomas Pilgrim J, Martinez Martínez JL, Martín Peñacoba R, González Tejón I, et al. Epidemiology of cardiovascular diseases and risk factors in primary care. Spanish Journal of Cardiology. 2015;

31. Celermajer DS, Chow CK, Marijon E, Anstey NM, Woo KS. Cardiovascular disease in the developing world: prevalences, patterns, and the potential of early disease detection. JACC. 2018;

32. Gibbons RJ, Balady GJ, Bridker JT et al. ACC/AHA 2016 guideline update for exercise testing: a report of the American College of Cardiology/American Heart Association Task Force on Practice guidelines, 2016 Disponible (http://www.acc.org/clinical/guidelines/ exercise/dirlndex.htm.2016).

33. Banka VS, Helfant RH. Temporal sequence of dynamic contractile characteristcs in ischemic and nonischemic myocardium after the coronary ligation. Am J Cardiol. 2016;

34. Celermajer DS, Chow CK, Marijon E, Anstey NM, Woo KS.Cardiovascular disease in the developing world: prevalences, patterns, an thepotential of early disease detection. JACC. 2018;

35. Filqueiras Ramas D,Juan Baguda J .Manual Chief Operating Officer Cardiology y cardiovascular medicine international 9th edition of Madrit CTO 2017.

36. Alvarez Syntheses R. Medicine General Comprehensive. The Havana: Medical Sciences; 2014; Vol. 4: Medicine and Health

37. Rock Goderich Mecina Internal. The Havana Medical Sciences 2017 I take II Medicine and Health

38. Days Villanueva Manual of heart disease in he patient old man .Madrit Medical Sciences 2018

39. Gibbons RJ, Balady GJ, bridker J.T. et. to the. ACC/AHA 2016 guideline update for exercise testing: a report of the American College of Cardiology/American Heart Association Task Force on Practice guidelines, 2016 Available (http://www.acc.org/clinical/guidelines/ exercise/dirlndex.htm.2016).
40. Albero Medrano. Incidence and prevalence of the heart disease ischemic .Rev Esp of Health Publish 2016
41. Artalejo Rodriguez .Congress of the diseases cardiovascular.Spanish Rev of Cardiology 2017

42. Brizuela.Guardiola.Cardiopathy ischemic to level primary rev Spanish cardiology

43. Ades PA. Cardiac rehabilitation and secondary prevention of coronary heart disease. N Engl J Med. 2016

44. Agati L, Majo F.D, Madonna M.P, Celani F, Funaro S, Tonti G. Assessment of myocardial viability in patients with postischemic left ventricular dysfunction: role of myocardial contrast echocardiography. Echocardiography. 2016

45. Rojo Cruz. Epidemiologia de las enfermedades Cardiovasculares.Medicina Preventiva ySalud Publica.2015

46. Gibbons RJ, Balady GJ, Bridker JT et al. ACC/AHA 2016 guideline update for exercise testing: a report of the American College of Cardiology/American Heart Association Task Force on Practice guidelines, 2016 Disponible (http://www.acc.org/clinical/guidelines/ exercise/dirlndex.htm.2016).

47. Marrugat J., García M., Elosua R., Aldasoro E., Tormo M.J., Zurriaga O., et al. Short-term (28 days) prognosis between genders according to the type of coronary event (Q-wave versus non–Q-wave acute myocardial infarction versus unstable angina pectoris). The American journal of cardiology. 2018

48. Marrugat J, Sala J, Masià R, Pavesi M, Sanz G, Valle V, et al. Mortality differences between men and women following first myocardial infarction. JAMA. 2016.

49. Sanz GA. Stratification of the risk in the syndromes coronary acute: an unsolved problem. Rev Esp Cardiol. 2017;

50. Savonittoa S, Moricib N, De Servic S. Treatment of coronary syndromes treble of seniors and patients with comorbidities. Rev Esp Cardiol. 2016;

51. Tahir SM, Price LL, Shah PB, Welt FG. Eighteen year (1985- 2016) analysis of incidence, mortality, and cardiac procedure outcomes of acute myocardial infarction in patients > or = 65 years of age. Am J Cardiol. 2016.

52. Viana Weaver, Ana. Evolution temporary of the treatment of the heart attack

Acute myocardial infarction in elderly patients and its impact on survival short and long term. Directed by Héctor Bueno and Francisco Fernández-Áviles. University Complutense of Madrid. Faculty of Medicine, 2018

53. wool, F., Bull, V., Cuts, R., Sanchez, TO. (2008). Interheart, a Case-control study on risk factors for Myocardial Infarction in the World and Latin America. Reflection on an original article. Magazine of the students of the Industrial University of Santander Medicas UIS. Available at: http://www.medicasuis.org/anteriores/volumen21.3/5.pdf

54. Reis E, Takao C. Zimmer A. Batista V, De Lima J, Leite A. Association of cardiovascular risk factors with the different presentations of acute coronary syndrome. Rev Latino-Am Enfermagem. [Online].2014. [Cited 03-16-2019], 22(4); 538-46. Available at: http://www.scielo.br/pdf/rlae/v22n4/es_0104-1169-rlae-22-04-00538.pd

55. Stack R, Rodriguez TO, Census G, Crag EITHER, Kwaku K. Heart attack of myocardium in the elderly. Comparative study. Annals of Cardiac and Vascular Surgery. 2016

56. Dr. Julia Tamara Alvarez Cuts, Dr. They lived Beautiful Hernandez, II Dr.Gipsy de los Ángeles Pérez Hechavarría, Dr. Orlando Antomarchi Duany I andDra. María Emilia Bolívar Carrión, Coronary risk factors associates to heart attack sharp of myocardium in he Elderly, MAGAZINE SCIELO- MEDISAN vol.17 no.1 Santiago of Cuba jan. 2016

57. Christopher J. O'Donnel and cabbage. Factors cardiovascular risk . Perspectives derived from the Framingham Heart Study. Spanish Journal of Cardiology. Vol. 61. No. 03. March 2008 Quintanar Guzmán A. (2010). Analysis of the quality of life in older adults in the municipality of Tetepango, Hidalgo through the whoqol-bref instrument. University Autonomous of the State of Gentleman. Thesis of undergraduate. Available at: http://www.uaeh.edu.mx/nuestro_alumnado/esc_sup/actopan/licenciat ura /Analisis%20de%20la%20calidad%20de%20vida.pdf

58. Rodríguez Daza, KD (2011). Old Age and Aging. Research Group on Physical Activity and Human Development. University of Rosary beads. School of Medicine and Sciences of the Health. Madrid: Ed. Díaz de Santos, 2018. Available at: http://www.urosario.edu.co/urosario_files/dd/dd857fc5-5a01-4355- b07a-e2f 0720b216b.pd

59. Alonso J., Well H., Bardaji TO., García-Moll X., Badia X., Layola M., Carreño A. Influence of sex on mortality and management of acute coronary syndrome in Spain. Rev Esp Cardiol. 2017;

60. Baena Diez J.M., of the Val Garcia J.L., Tomas Pelegrina J, Martínez Martínez JL, Martín Peñacoba R, González Tejón I, et al. Epidemiology of cardiovascular

diseases and risk factors in attention primary. Magazine Spanish of Cardiology. 2015

61. Banegas J.R., Villar F, Graciani TO, Rodríguez-Artalejo F. Epidemiology of cardiovascular diseases in Spain Rev Esp Cardiol Supl. 2016

62. Brahmajee K, Pharoah PO, Ventava SK... Reperfusion therapy in Myocardial infarction. Am J Pulic Health. 2003;

63. Andrew SAY, Lamb A, Magána P, Joy SAY, Leon M, Luengo SAY, etc al. Long-term mortality and hospital readmission after acute myocardial infarction: a study of follow-up of eight years. Rev Esp Cardiol. 2012;

64. Avezum A, Makdisse M, Spencer F, Gore JM, Fox KA, Montalescot G, et al. Impact of age on management and outcome of acute coronary syndrome: observations from the Global Registry of Acute Coronary Events. American Heart Journal. 2015;

65. Banka VS, Helfant RH. Temporal sequence of dynamic contractile characteristcs in ischemic and nonischemic myocardium after the coronary ligation. Am J Cardiol. 1974; 34: 158-162

66. Bauer T, Koeth O, Junger C, Heer T, Wienbergen H, Gitt A, et al. Effect of an invasive strategy on in-hospital outcome in elderly patients with non-STelevation myocardial infarction. European heart Journal. 2017;

67. Delcan JL. Ischemic heart disease. Epidemiology of Ischemic Heart Disease: Factors of Risk and Prevention Primary. Madrid: Salvat editions; 2006

68. Sanz GA. Stratification of the risk in the syndromes coronary acute: an unsolved problem. Rev Esp Cardiol. 2018

69. Dr. José Antonio González Pompa et al. Risk factors for the occurrence of acute myocardial infarction in smoking patients. Hospital General academic "Carlos Manuel of "Cespedes" Bayamo. Granma, Cuba

70. MayUS Dept of Health and Human Services. The Health Benefits of Smoking Cessation.A report of the Surgeon General. USDHHS, Centers for Disease Control. Office of Smoking and Health; 1990.DHHS Publication (CDC) 2017-2018

71. Serrano M, Madoz E, Ezpeleta I, San Julián B, Amezqueta C, Pérez Marco JA. Abandonment of the tobacco and risk of new heart attack in coronary patients: nested case-control study. Rev Esp Cardiol 2016

72. Castle L; Lycea M. Dyslipoproteinemia and diabetes mellitus. Rev Cuban CardiolCirCardiovasc 2016

73. Velázquez-Monroy O, Rosas Peralta M, Lara Esqueda A, Pastelín Hernández G, Castle W, Attie F, et al. Prevalence It is interrelationship in chronic non-

communicable diseases and cardiovascular risk factors in Mexico: results finals of the Survey National Health Service (ENSA) 2000. Arch Cardiol Mex. 2008

74. Gonzalez Maqueda YO. Hypertension arterial and heart disease ischemic . Rev.Esp. Cardio. 2018;

75. Bertomeu V, Quiles J. The hypertension in attention primary: Do we know the magnitude of the problem and act accordingly? Rev Esp Cardiol. 2017

76. Lamb TO, Dark J, Happiness AND. Hypertension arterial and metabolic syndrome. Rev Esp Cardiol. 2016

77. Mancia G, Laurent S, Agabiti-Rosei E, Ambrosioni E, Burniere M, Caulfieldf MJ, et al. Reappraisal of European guidelines on hypertension management: a European Society of Hypertension Task Force document. J Hypertens. 2019

78. López F, Cortés M. 72 . Mancia G, Laurent S, Agabiti-Rosei E, Ambrosioni E, Burniere M, Caulfieldf MJ, et al. Reappraisal of European guidelines on hypertension management: a European Society of Hypertension Task Force document. J Hypertens. 2019 Obesidad y corazón. RevEsp Cardiol.2019

79. Hastie CE, Padmanabhan S, Slack R, Pell AC, Oldroyd KG, Flapan AD, et al. Obesity paradox in a cohort of 4880 consecutive patients undergoing percutaneous coronary intervention. Eur Heart J 2018

80. Edelsio Dorta Rodriguez; 1 Robert Javier Tablada Ramirez; 2 Aracelis of the Charity Arias Jimenez. Factors of risk heart attack sharp of the myocardium in patients diagnosed with arterial hypertension. Multimed. Medical Magazine. Granma 2017

81. Gonzalez Ramirez. Adherence index to dietary hygiene measures in patients with heart disease ischemic Magazine Medical. Veracruz 2016

82. Ahern, D. K., Gorkin, L., & Anderson, J. L. (2001). Biobehavioral variables and mortality or cardiac arrest in the Cardiac Arrhythmia Pilot Study (CAPS). American Journal of Cardiology, 66, 59-62.

83. Álvarez A, Rodríguez L, Chacón T. Risk factors for cardiomyopathy hypertensive. Rev Cuban Med 2016 (accessed 12 May 2016);46(1). Available at:http : //scielo.sld . cu/scielo.php?script=sci_arttex t &pid=S0034-75232007000100003&lng=es&nrm=iso&tlng=es

84. Velázquez-Monroy O, Rosas Peralta M, Lara Esqueda A, Pastelín Hernández G, Castle C, Attie F, et to the. Prevalence and interrelationship of chronic non-communicable diseases and risk factors cardiovascular in Mexico: results finals of the Survey National Health Service (ENSA) 2000. Arch Cardiol Mex. 20018

85. Dr. Cisneros Sánchez, Factors of risk of the heart disease ischemic Cuban

Journal of Comprehensive General Medicine Havana 2013

86. Days Eagle Characterization of the factors of risk vascular in adult patients CorSalud 2018 Villa Clara Cuba

87. Alfonso Alfonso Characterization of the factors of irrigation in patients with chronic heart disease Rev. Med Electron 2017 Sagua la Grande

88. Society Spanish of Cardiology. The race conditions he cardiovascular risk RevEsp Cardiol.2019

89. Castro Gutierrez heart disease ischemic shapes clinics and MEDICIEGO 2015 complications

90. Delcán, JL Ischemic Cardiopathy. Epidemiology of Ischemic Heart Disease: Factors of Risk and Prevention Primary. Madrid 2018.

91. Royo Ma, Wolves J.M. he state of the prevention cardiovascular in Spain.Medicine Clinic [Internet].2016 available in http://udaceba.cat. One.cu.sld./. wepet content/uploads/ 2018

92. Nelson DE, Kinkerdall RS, Lawton RL et al. Surveillance for smoking- attributable mortality and years of potential life lost; by state United States, 2016 MMWR CDC 2016

93. Blumel MJE, Prieto DJC, Loyal ITEM. Impact of the factors of coronary risk in middle-aged women. Rev. Méd Chile. 2018

94. Andrew AND, Lion M, Lamb TO, Magallon R, Magan Q, Later AND, et to the. Cardiovascular risk factors and lifestyle associated with the appearance early of heart attack sharp of myocardium. RevEspCardiol. 2017

95. Roka Ivanova Giorgeva .Factors of risk cardiovascular .Editorial university of Granada .Rev ESp 2018

96. Santos C, Badimón J. High-density lipoproteins and risk reduction cardiovascular: promises either realities? RevEspCardiol. 2017

97. Chapman J.M., Goerke LS,.Dixon W. Measuring the risks of coronary heart disease in adult population groups.Public Health 2017

98. Guallar Q, Gil M, Lion I, Graciani TO, Bayan TO, Taboada J, et to the. Magnitude and management of hypercholesterolemia in the adult population of Spain, 2008-2010: the ENRICA study. RevEspCardiol. 2017

99. Dr. Jaromir Ramon Shepherdess Benavides Thesis doctoral. Factors of Risk Associated with Acute Coronary Syndrome in the HEODRA Department of Internal Medicine. Available at: http://hera.ugr.es/tesisugr/15888794.pdf (accessed May 12 2017).

100. Masterson R, Smeeth L, Gilman R, Miranda J. Physical activity and cardiovascular risk factors among rural and urban groups and rural-to- urban migrants in Peru: a cross-sectional study. Rev PanamSaludPublica 2017[citado 2017Mar21].Disponible en:http://www.scielosp.org/pdf/rpsp/v28n1/v28n1a01.pdf 48

101. Dr.:Katherine Lisbet Vilchez Cabrera .Thesis doctoral Behavior of risk factors associated with acute coronary syndrome Available: www.sac.org.ar/rac/2003/v4_b/cg-1.pdf

Board 1

Distribution of Adults greater with heart disease (cases) according to age and sex. Medical Office 8. Manacas health area. 2019-2020

Age	Adults Greater with Ischemic heart disease (Cases)					
	Male		Female		TOTAL	
	No.	%	No.	%	No.	%
‹65 a70 YEARS	4	11.7	3	8.82	7	20.5
Elderly 70 YEARS	17	fifty	10	29.4	27	79.5
Total	twenty-one	61.7	13	38.2	3. 4	100

Board 2

Distribution of Adults greater with heart disease (cases) depending on color of the skin. Medical Office 8. Manacas health area. 2019-2020

Color of the fur	No.	%
White	25	73.52
No white	9	26.47
Total	3. 4	100

Board 3

Distribution of older adults with heart disease (cases) according to type of heart disease Medical Office 8. Manacas health area. 2019-2020

Guy of heart disease	No.	%
Angina	16	47.05
Insufficiency cardiac	eleven	32.35
Syndrome acute coronary	7	20.58
Total	3. 4	100

Board 4

Distribution of older adults with heart disease (cases) according to first-degree family history of pathology. Medical Office 8. Manacas health area. 2019-2020

APF of Ischemic Heart Disease in first degree relative	Cluster cases		Control group		OR
	No	%	No	%	
With APF	29	85.2	18	52.9	5.1
Without APF	5	14.7	16	47.0	
Total	3. 4	100	3. 4	100	

Board 5

Distribution of Adults greater with heart disease (cases) according to he habit of smoke. Medical Office 8. Manacas health area. 2019-2020

Habit of smoking	Cases Group		Control group		OR
	No	%	No	%	
Smoker	28	82.35	23	67.34	2.23
Non smoker	6	17.64	eleven	32.35	
Total	3. 4	100	3. 4	100	

Board 6

Distribution of older adults with heart disease (cases) according to personal pathological history of diabetes mellitus. Medical Office 8. Manacas health area. 2019-202

Mellitus diabetes	Cluster cases		Control group		OR
	No	%	No	%	
With APP of Mellitus diabetes	18	52.94	3	8.82	12.3
Without APP of diabetes mellitus	16	47.05	31	91.17	
Total	3. 4	100	3. 4	100	

Board 7

Distribution of older adults with heart disease (cases) according to personal pathological history of high blood pressure. Medical Office 8. Manacas health area. 2019-202

APP Arterial hypertension	Cluster cases		Control group		OR
	No	%	No	%	
With APP	33	97.05	twenty	58.82	23.1
Without APP	1	2.94	14	41.17	
Total	3. 4	100	3. 4	100	

Board 8

Distribution of older adults with heart disease (cases) according to personal pathological history of dyslipidemia. Medical Office 8. Manacas health area. 2019-2021

Dyslipidemia	Cluster cases		Control group		OR
	No	%	No	%	
With dyslipidemia	28	82.35	8	23.52	
No dyslipidemia	6	17.64	26	76.47	15.1
Total	3. 4	100	3. 4	100	

Board 9

Distribution of older adults with heart disease (cases) according to personal pathological history of obesity. Medical Office 8. Manacas health area. 2019-2021

APP Obesity	Cluster Cases		Control group		OR
	No	%	No	%	
With APP	32	94.11	24	70.58	6.66
Without APP	2	5.88	10	2.94	
Total	3. 4	100	3. 4	100	

Exhibit 1

***Informed Consent** POLYCLINIC ACADEMIC MANACA SANTO DOMINGO.*
I:I have been informed of the importance of morbidity and mortality due to ischemic heart disease in the population of the older adult of CMF No. 8 of the Manacas health area, which currently represent a serious problem of health so does necessary to collect information about them and raise the state of knowledge of their prevention and management to improve health status of this population. The study that HE will make be through of anonymous questionnaires and information collection will only be employed with investigative purposes, so I declare to be informed of the objective as well as having received an explanation of the usefulness of the research. I have been informed that if I do not cooperate with the study, this will not represent problems for me and my attention from the health personnel .

And so that the above is recorded, this document is signed in Manacas to the days, of the month of 20

IC:
Signature

Exhibit 2

Interview

1- *You Smoke either used to smoke?*
2- *That Time was smoking?*
3- *That number of cigarettes smoke either HE used to smoke diary?*
4- *In his home either work smoke?*
5- *You presents frequently infections respiratory low?*
6- *How many times to the year?*

Exhibit 3

Guide of revision of medical records

-Age when getting sick.
-Background pathological personal of hypertension arterial, of diabetes mellitus, from dyslipidemia
-Background pathological relatives of first line.
-Index of mass bodily

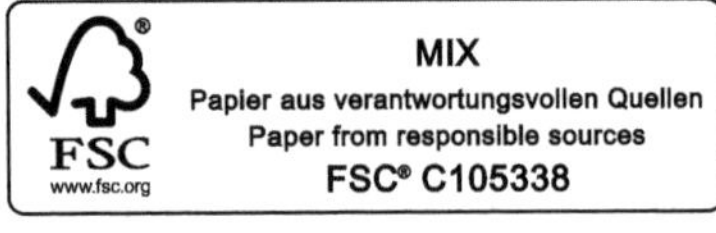

Printed by Books on Demand GmbH, Norderstedt / Germany